COMPACT GUIDES TO FITNESS & HEALTH

8 WAYS TO LOWER YOUR RISK OF A HEART ATTACK OR STROKE

CONTENT PROVIDED BY MAYO CLINIC HEALTH INFORMATION

MASON CREST PUBLISHERS
Philadelphia, Pennsylvania

8 Ways to Lower Your Risk of a Heart Attack or Stroke provides reliable, practical, easy-to-understand information on living a longer and healthier life. Much of the information comes directly from the experience of Mayo Clinic physicians, nurses, registered dietitians, health educators and other health care professionals. This book supplements the advice of your personal physician, whom you should consult for individual medical problems. MAYO, MAYO CLINIC, MAYO CLINIC HEALTH INFORMATION and the Mayo triple-shield logo are marks of Mayo Foundation for Medical Education and Research.

Hardcover Library Edition Published 2002
Mason Crest Publishers
370 Reed Road
Suite 302
Broomall, PA 19008-0914
(866) MCP-BOOK (toll free)

First Printing
1 2 3 4 5 6 7 8 9 10
Library of Congress Cataloging-in-Publication Data on file at the Library of Congress

ISBN 1-59084-246-4 (hc)
Printed in the United States of America

Contents

It's time to change your lifestyle 4

Strategy 1:
Don't smoke 6

Strategy 2:
Limit fat and cholesterol 10

Strategy 3:
Exercise daily 15

Strategy 4:
Maintain a healthy weight 18

Strategy 5:
Eat more fiber 23

Strategy 6:
Eat more foods with antioxidants . . 26

Strategy 7:
Watch your blood pressure 28

Strategy 8:
Manage stress 30

Photos on cover and pages 10, 32 © PhotoDisc Inc. Photos on pages 6,
14, 15, 18, 23, 27, 28, 30 © Corel Corporation. Photo on page 16 ©
Mayo Clinic. Photo on page 26 © Stockbyte.

8 ways to lower your risk of a heart attack or stroke

It's time to change your lifestyle

You can't turn back the clock or reconfigure your family tree to lower your risk of a heart attack or stroke. Age and genetics are powerful, unchangeable predictors of coronary artery disease and stroke.

Coronary artery disease is the narrowing of the arteries that serve your heart. You have a heart attack when one of these arteries becomes blocked — usually by a blood clot — cutting off the supply of oxygen and nutrients to your heart. Stroke, another common and deadly form of cardiovascular disease, occurs when the blood supply to your brain is disrupted. This can be caused by a blockage or a rupture in the arteries supplying oxygen and other nutrients to your brain.

However, research continues to point out how a healthy lifestyle can improve and, in some cases, eliminate many significant risk factors for coronary artery disease and stroke. These risk factors include smoking, high blood pressure, obesity, diabetes, and undesirable levels of cholesterol and triglycerides.

Because control of coronary artery disease and stroke is evolving, it's too soon to make definite recommendations about all issues related to lifestyle. Yet this booklet offers eight sound strategies you can adopt now to reduce your risks and improve the quality of your life.

Atherosclerosis

When excess cholesterol is in your blood, cholesterol-containing fatty deposits can accumulate in your arteries — a process called atherosclerosis. As these deposits build up, blood flow is reduced — putting you at risk of heart attack or stroke.

Many of the strategies in this booklet can help you reduce your risk of atherosclerosis.

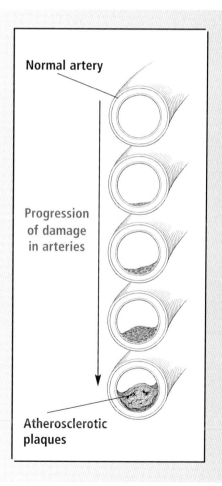

Normal artery

Progression of damage in arteries

Atherosclerotic plaques

Strategy 1:
Don't smoke

Tobacco smoke contains more than 4,000 chemi-
cals. Many of these substances can damage your
heart and the blood vessels that supply your
heart and brain. Not smoking is the single best
thing you can do to reduce your risk of a heart
attack or stroke.

Extensive damage

Smoking damages the walls of your blood vessels,
making them prone to the buildup of cholesterol-
containing fatty deposits called plaques — a
condition known as atherosclerosis. Smoking
may also reduce the proportion of high-density
lipoprotein (HDL) cholesterol to low-density
lipoprotein (LDL) cholesterol in your blood. High
blood levels of LDL ("bad") cholesterol increase
your risk of atherosclerosis. In contrast, high levels of HDL ("good") cholesterol are protective
because they may prevent formation of plaques.

In addition, nicotine in cigarette smoke makes
your heart work harder by constricting blood
vessels and increasing your heart rate and blood
pressure. Carbon monoxide in cigarette smoke
replaces some of the oxygen in your blood. This
also increases blood pressure by forcing your
heart to work harder to supply adequate oxygen.

Why quit?

If you smoke cigarettes, your risk of a heart attack or stroke is at least double that of non-smokers. And the risk increases with the number of cigarettes you smoke each day. Cigars, pipes and chewing tobacco also increase your risk, but to a lesser degree.

When you quit, your risk of coronary artery disease drops dramatically within 1 to 2 years. Ten years after quitting, your risk of a stroke is about the same as that of a nonsmoker.

Adopting the right approach

It takes most people three to four attempts to stop smoking permanently. However, each try increases your chances of success. Think of each relapse not as a failure but as an opportunity to learn. In this way, you can avoid or change the circumstances leading to relapse.

There's no single best way to quit smoking. However, you're most likely to be successful if you plan ahead:

• *Commit to quitting* — List all of the positive reasons you want to stop smoking. Then be sure you're ready to follow through on your commitment.

• *Set a date* — Mark the calendar for 2 weeks to 1 month from now. Try to avoid a time when other factors may increase stress in your life. But be realistic. There's no ideal day to quit.

• *Devise a plan* — Identify trigger behaviors such as drinking coffee or talking on the phone. Decide how to change your response to these situations. Taking a walk and eating a healthy snack are possible distractions.

• *Condition yourself* — If you smoke two packs a day, wean yourself to one. Don't buy a new pack until you finish the present one. Switch to a brand you don't enjoy as much.

• *Seek support* — Ask someone to exercise with you or call regularly with words of encouragement. Refusing the help of others protects the addiction, not you. For heavy addiction, consider counseling, a support group or an inpatient program.

Dangers of secondhand smoke

Cigarettes are bad for you even if you don't smoke.

In the United States, experts estimate that more than 50,000 nonsmokers die each year from exposure to secondhand tobacco smoke. If you breathe it regularly, you're probably at risk. Consider these facts:

• Exposure to secondhand smoke causes about 30 times as many lung cancer deaths as all regulated air pollutants combined.

• A 1996 study of 32,000 nurses found that regular exposure to secondhand smoke doubles a woman's risk of a heart attack.

• Secondhand smoke leads to coughing, phlegm, chest discomfort, reduced lung function, and red, itchy, watery eyes.

- *Think positively* — Stay focused by reviewing your list of reasons for quitting. Then take it one day at a time.

Cigarette substitutes

Research shows that medications can help people gradually withdraw from nicotine and stop smoking. Talk with your doctor or pharmacist about the options below, including side effects.

Nicotine replacement products

Patch — Available without a prescription, you apply these patches to an area of skin to provide a steady dose of absorbed nicotine. As you lower the patch dose, the nicotine levels decrease. Ask your doctor or pharmacist about the recommended length of treatment.

Nasal spray — Available by prescription only, you spray nicotine directly into each nostril. Typical length of therapy is 6 to 12 weeks.

Gum — To use this over-the-counter product, chew it a few times, then let it sit between your cheek and gum. The nicotine is absorbed through the lining of your mouth. Gradually decrease use and stop altogether in 3 to 6 months.

Inhaler — Available by prescription, the inhaler is a plastic cylinder about the size of a cigarette. Inside the cylinder is a cartridge with nicotine. When you puff on the device, nicotine vapors are absorbed through the lining of your mouth. Usual length of therapy is 6 to 12 weeks.

Non-nicotine medication

Bupropion (Zyban) — Bupropion is a non-nicotine antidepressant that's marketed under the name Zyban to help people stop smoking. Treatment is usually 7 to 12 weeks. Bupropion is also marketed under the name Wellbutrin for the treatment of depression. Don't use more than one form of bupropion at a time. Don't use bupropion if you've recently taken a monoamine oxidase inhibitor (MAOI, an antidepressant) or if you have a history of seizures, head trauma, stroke, anorexia or bulimia. Bupropion may cause high blood pressure in a small percentage of people, especially if used with the nicotine patch, so periodic blood pressure checks are important. If you have high blood pressure, heart disease, kidney or liver disease, or you regularly drink alcohol or take benzodiazepines (Valium, Librium, Xanax, others), ask your doctor about the risks of using bupropion. Excessive use of alcohol or abrupt withdrawal from alcohol while using bupropion may increase the risk of seizure.

Strategy 2:
Limit fat and cholesterol

A diet high in cholesterol and fat, especially saturated fat, promotes atherosclerosis (the buildup of plaques in blood vessels) by increasing the amount of fat and cholesterol in your blood. Although medications may improve blood cholesterol levels, a combination of sound nutrition and regular exercise is your first line of defense.

Two basic steps

Changes in your diet, along with exercise, may reduce your total blood cholesterol level by up to 15 percent. (See "What do your cholesterol and triglyceride levels mean?" on page 24.)

What's the story on fish?

Fish may protect against coronary artery disease because it contains a type of polyunsaturated fat called omega-3 fatty acids. These fats may help improve HDL ("good") cholesterol and triglyceride levels. They also may help lower blood pressure slightly.

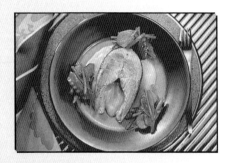

Omega-3 fatty acids occur naturally in cold-water fish — particularly salmon, mackerel, and albacore and white tuna. Eating these types of fish once or twice a week as part of a low-fat diet may reduce your risk of dying of coronary artery disease. However, eating lots of fish — five or six servings a week (one serving is about 3 ounces) — doesn't seem to provide any additional protection.

To improve your diet:

1. *Reduce total fat to no more than 30 percent of your daily calories.* Limit all types of fat (see "Fats: The good and the bad" on page 14), but limit saturated fat to less than 10 percent of your calories. If you have high LDL ("bad") cholesterol or cardiovascular disease, limit saturated fat to less than 7 percent of daily calories. See the chart below to estimate your fat limits.

Calculate your fat limits	Daily calorie level	Total fat grams (30% of calories)
Many women and older adults	1,600	53
Children, teen girls, active women, most men	2,200	73
Teen boys, active men	2,800	93

Some evidence suggests that monounsaturated fats, found in foods such as olive oil, walnuts and almonds, help lower LDL cholesterol levels. How-ever, monounsaturated fats — like all fats — have more than twice as many calories in a gram as carbohydrates or protein (9 vs. 4 calories). For most people, the best way to improve blood cholesterol levels is by losing weight through control of calories from all fats.

2. *Reduce dietary cholesterol.* Set your daily limit for dietary cholesterol at 300 milligrams or less. All foods made from animals contain cholesterol. Concentrated sources include organ meats, red meats, egg yolks, butter, whole milk and whole-milk cheeses. (See "Your low-fat, low-cholesterol eating guide," pages 12 to 13.)

Your low-fat, low-cholesterol eating guide

Here's a guide to help you keep fat within 30 percent of your total calories and cholesterol to less than 300 milligrams daily.

Make "Preferred" foods the basis of your diet. These foods are either fat- and cholesterol-free or low in fat and cholesterol.*

Food (Groups)	Preferred
Fruits and vegetables *5 or more daily servings*	Any fresh, frozen, canned or dried (Remember that canned foods are high in sodium.)
Grains (breads, cereals, rice, pasta) *6 to 11 daily servings*	Whole-grain breads and cereals, bagels, breadsticks, English muffins, brown rice, pasta, plain popcorn, pretzels, low-fat crackers
Dairy products (milk, yogurt, cheese) *2 to 3 daily servings*	Fat-free or low-fat (1%) milk, fat-free yogurt, fat-free and low-fat cheeses
Meat, poultry, fish, beans *2 to 3 daily servings* *(no more than 6 ounces of meat a day)*	Lean meats, fish and poultry without skin; dried beans, lentils; egg whites or egg substitutes; water-packed tuna or salmon; low-fat luncheon meats; low-fat hot dogs
Fats and oils *Use sparingly*	Monounsaturated oils (canola, olive, peanut), polyunsaturated oils (corn, safflower, sunflower, soybean, sesame, cottonseed), tub margarine, salad dressings with unsaturated oils

* Low-fat means no more than 3 grams of fat per serving. Low-cholesterol means no more than 20 milligrams of cholesterol and no more than 2 grams of saturated fat per serving. Check the label.

Limit "Occasional" foods to once or twice daily, and eat small portions. These foods have moderate amounts of fat or cholesterol. If you eat "Infrequent" foods at all, keep portions small and limit them to once or twice a week. These foods are highest in fat or cholesterol.

Occasional	Infrequent
Avocado, olives	Coconut; fruits and vegetables in cheese, cream, butter or heavy sauces; fried vegetables
Egg noodles, refined grains such as white bread and white rice	Croissants, muffins, regular snack crackers and chips, biscuits
Reduced-fat milk (2%), part-skim milk cheeses (mozzarella, ricotta, farmer), low-fat yogurt, ice milk, creamed cottage cheese (4%)	Whole milk, whole-milk yogurt and cheese, ice cream (regular and gourmet)
Shrimp, oysters, oil-packed fish, peanut butter, nuts, egg yolks	Organ meats, fatty and heavily marbled meats, spare ribs, cold cuts, hot dogs, sausage, bacon, fried meats
Creamy salad dressing, mayonnaise, reduced-fat sour cream and cream cheese, stick margarine	Shortening, lard, butter, cream, half-and-half, sour cream, cream cheese, gravy, most nondairy creamers, bacon fat, cream sauces, coconut oil, palm and palm kernel oils, cocoa butter (found in chocolate)

Fats: The good and the bad

Saturated fat: Raises blood cholesterol and increases the risk of coronary artery disease. *Found in:* Red meats, most dairy products, and coconut, palm and other tropical oils.

Polyunsaturated fat: Helps lower blood cholesterol but also seems to be susceptible to oxidation. (Oxidation enables cells in your arteries to absorb fats and cholesterol, speeding the buildup of artery-clogging plaques.) *Found in:* Vegetable oils such as safflower, corn, sunflower, soy and cottonseed oil.

Monounsaturated fat: Helps lower blood cholesterol and is more resistant to oxidation. *Found in:* Olive, canola and nut oils.

Trans fat (partially hydrogenated vegetable oil): Raises blood cholesterol and increases the risk of coronary artery disease. *Found in:* Stick margarine and shortening, which are often used in making cookies, crackers, candy bars and other prepared foods.

The soy burger is back

If your total cholesterol is greater than 250 mg/dL, substituting at least 25 grams of soy protein for animal protein daily may help lower cholesterol and triglyceride levels. One 3-ounce soy burger and 2 cups of soy milk contain about 30 grams of soy protein. (See "What do your cholesterol and triglyceride levels mean?" on page 22.)

Soybeans provide plentiful amounts of fiber. And even though soybeans contain moderate amounts of fat, their oils are primarily unsaturated. Most soy products also contain substances called isoflavones and phytoestrogens. Researchers suspect these plant hormones may lower blood cholesterol.

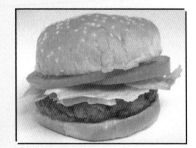

Adding soy to your diet may not eliminate your need for medication if you take a cholesterol-lowering drug. But substituting low-fat soy products for some animal protein as part of a low-fat diet is reasonable.

Strategy 3:
Exercise daily

If you exercise regularly, your overall risk of a heart attack is about half that of people who are sedentary and out of shape.

Regular exercise reduces risk of death from all causes, including heart disease and cancer. With routine exercise, you may reach a level of physical fitness comparable to an inactive person 10 to 20 years younger.

How exercise promotes longevity
Regular exercise may help you live longer by:

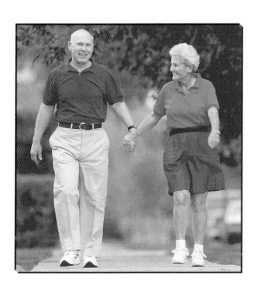

- Increasing the size of your coronary arteries and reducing atherosclerosis

- Decreasing the level of cholesterol in your blood

- Lowering blood pressure slightly

- Helping to control weight

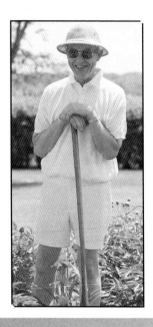

Key is frequency, not intensity

To condition your heart safely, follow these guidelines:

- *Intensity* — Choose moderate-intensity activities. Moderate activity is comparable to the effort you exert during a brisk walk. (See chart below.)

- *Frequency* — Try to be moderately active on most, if not all, days.

- *Duration* — Aim to burn 200 calories a day by spending 30 to 40 minutes in any combination of moderate-intensity activities.

Activity	Calories burned in 10 minutes of activity*
• Brisk walking • Golfing (walk, don't ride)	50 to 60
• Hoeing the garden • Leisurely bike ride (less than 10 mph)	60 to 70
• Playing tennis • Scrubbing the kitchen floor	70 to 80
• Swimming (slow crawl)	80 to 90

*Calories are based on a 150-pound person. If you weigh less than 150 pounds, you need to spend more time to burn the same number of calories. Weighing more than 150 pounds means you burn the same number of calories in less time.

Is exercise risky?

Most heart attacks occur during rest — not activity. Of people who have heart attacks during strenuous exertion, most are sedentary, have underlying heart disease and overdo it.

To minimize risks and maximize benefits of exercise, check with your doctor for recommendations if you're over 40, out of shape, or if you have a chronic condition such as cardiovascular disease or diabetes. Then follow these tips:

- *Exercise regularly* — Cardiovascular risk rises if you alternate intense workouts with weeks to months of inactivity.

- *Warm up and cool down* — This reduces stress on your heart and risk of muscle strain.

- *Exercise, don't compete* — Avoid physical and emotional intensity in competitive sports.

- *Wait 2 to 3 hours after a large meal before exercising* — Digestion directs blood to your digestive system and away from your heart.

- *Take the talk test* — If you can talk easily while exercising, you're probably not overexerting.

- *Tailor exercise to the weather* — Reduce speed and distance when it's hot and humid.

- *Avoid start-and-stop activities* — Control physical exertion with a continuous form of exercise, such as walking or cycling.

- *Don't walk or jog near heavy traffic* — Carbon monoxide pollution reduces oxygen supply to your heart.

- *Listen to your body* — If you have dizziness, nausea, weakness, chest pain or shortness of breath, stop exercising and seek medical attention.

Strategy 4:
Maintain a healthy weight

Being overweight makes you more likely to have high blood pressure, cardiovascular disease or diabetes.

Losing weight through diet and exercise may help reduce your risk of a heart attack or stroke by lowering blood pressure and improving cholesterol levels.

What is a healthy weight?
Consider your weight healthy if:

• You don't have a medical problem that's caused or aggravated by your weight.

• You don't have a family history of a weight-related condition.

• Your weight falls within the recommended limits for healthy weight.

The Dietary Guidelines for Americans bases recommendations for healthy weight on the body-mass index (BMI). The link between this indirect measure of your body fat and risk of death provides the recommended limits for weight. (To figure your BMI and determine your obesity-related risk of disease, see "Does your weight put you at risk?" on pages 20 to 22.)

Losing weight safely and permanently
If you need to lose weight, here's how to improve your chances of getting rid of the pounds for good:

- *Make a commitment* — Lose weight because you want to, not because you want to please others. Become self-motivated.

- *Get your priorities straight* — It takes a lot of mental and physical energy to change your habits. Plan to lose weight when you aren't distracted by any major problems or commitments.

- *Set a realistic goal* — Try to achieve a comfortable weight, for example, one you maintained easily as a young adult. If you've always been overweight, you may not need to lose as much weight as you think to improve your blood pressure, energy, and levels of cholesterol and blood sugar.

- *Don't starve yourself* — Cutting calories to less than 1,400 doesn't allow enough food to be satisfying in the long term. Eating fewer than 1,200 calories makes it difficult to get adequate amounts of some nutrients. It also promotes temporary loss of fluids rather than permanent loss of fat. To lose body fat slowly and safely, figure:

$$\underline{\hspace{3cm}} \text{ x } 10 \text{ } = \text{ } \underline{\hspace{3cm}}$$
(current weight in pounds)   **(daily calories)**

This calorie goal should help you lose about 1 to 2 pounds a week.

- *Get and stay active* — The best way to lose body fat is through steady exercise lasting longer than 20 minutes. But any extra movement helps burn calories and reduces your overall risk of a heart attack or stroke.

Does your weight put you at risk?

STEP 1: Figure your body mass index (BMI).

BMI is a more valuable measurement of body fat and health risks than your bathroom scale or weight-for-height tables. Higher BMI numbers are associated with higher blood fats and blood pressure and an increased risk of certain diseases, such as cardiovascular disease, stroke, diabetes and some cancers. To calculate your BMI, use the chart below. Find your height in the left column, then locate your weight. Your BMI is the number at the top of that column. (See example below.)

BODY MASS INDEX								
	19	**20**	**21**	**22**	**23**	**24**	**25**	**26**
HEIGHT					WEIGHT (pounds)			
4' 10"	91	96	100	105	110	115	119	124
4' 11"	94	99	104	109	114	119	124	128
5' 0"	97	102	107	112	118	123	128	133
5' 1"	100	106	111	116	122	127	132	137
5' 2"	104	109	115	120	126	131	136	142
5' 3"	107	113	118	124	130	135	141	146
5' 4"	110	116	122	128	134	140	145	151
5' 5"	114	120	126	132	138	144	150	156
5' 6"	118	124	130	136	142	148	155	161
5' 7"	121	127	134	140	146	153	159	166
5' 8"	125	131	138	144	151	158	164	171
5' 9"	128	135	142	149	155	162	169	176
5' 10"	132	139	146	153	160	167	174	181
5' 11"	136	143	150	157	165	172	179	186
6' 0"	140	147	154	162	169	177	184	191
6' 1"	144	151	159	166	174	182	189	197
6' 2"	148	155	163	171	179	184	194	202
6' 3"	152	160	168	176	184	192	200	208
6' 4"	156	164	172	180	189	197	205	213

The BMI is a good but not perfect guide. For example, muscle weighs more than fat, and many people who are very muscular and physically fit have high BMIs without added health risks. The BMI is not appropriate if you're pregnant.

• If your BMI falls below 18.5, you're underweight.

• If your BMI falls between 18.5 and 24.9, you're in the healthy range, and this suggests that you don't need to lose weight. But Asians with a BMI over 23 could be at risk of health problems.

continued

BODY MASS INDEX								
27	**28**	**29**	**30**	**31**	**32**	**33**	**34**	**35**
WEIGHT (pounds)								
129	134	138	143	148	153	158	162	167
133	138	143	148	153	158	163	168	173
138	143	148	153	158	163	168	174	179
143	148	153	158	164	169	174	180	185
147	153	158	164	169	175	180	186	191
152	158	163	169	175	180	186	191	197
157	163	169	174	180	186	192	197	204
162	168	174	180	186	192	198	204	210
167	173	179	186	192	198	204	210	216
172	178	185	191	198	204	211	217	223
177	184	190	197	203	210	216	223	230
182	189	196	203	209	216	223	230	236
188	194	202	209	216	222	229	236	243
193	200	208	215	222	229	236	243	250
199	206	213	221	228	235	242	250	258
204	212	219	227	235	242	250	257	265
210	218	225	233	241	249	256	264	272
216	224	232	240	248	256	264	272	279
221	230	238	246	254	263	271	279	287

- If your BMI falls between 25 and 29.9, you're overweight.

- If your BMI is 30 or higher, you're obese.

STEP 2: Measure your waist.

Using the body mass index and waist circumference as guides, the table below helps assess risk of obesity-related diseases.

Measure your waist at your navel. For men with a BMI of 25 or greater, a waist circumference of 40 inches or more is associated with higher risk of weight-related diseases. For women with a BMI of 25 or greater, a waist circumference of 35 inches or more is associated with higher risks.

Does your weight put you at risk of high blood pressure, cardiovascular disease and type 2 diabetes?

	Body mass index (BMI)*	Waist measurement: Men: Less than 40 inches Women: Less than 35 inches	Waist measurement: Men: 40 inches or more Women: 35 inches or more
Overweight	25 to 29.9	Increased risk	High risk
Obese	30 to 34.9	High risk	Very high risk
	35 to 39.9	Very high risk	Very high risk
Extremely obese	40 or over	Extremely high risk	Extremely high risk

*If your BMI is between 18.5 and 24.9, your weight is not likely to have a major effect on your health. If your BMI is 25 or more, you're at increased risk of serious health problems. Asians with a BMI over 23 may have an increased risk of health problems.

Strategy 5:
Eat more fiber

Grains, legumes (lentils and dried peas and beans), fruits and vegetables contain two types of dietary fiber — insoluble and soluble.

Insoluble fiber, found mainly in whole grains, helps prevent constipation and diverticulosis and possibly reduces your risk of colon cancer.

Soluble fiber, contained in oats, dried beans, and fruits such as apples, oranges and grapefruit, may help lower blood cholesterol. (See "Fiber figures," page 25.)

How much benefit can you expect?

One widely accepted theory for soluble fiber's benefits is its ability to bind to cholesterol in your intestinal tract. When passed in your stool, fiber takes cholesterol with it, lowering cholesterol levels in your blood.

The cholesterol-lowering effects, however, are modest. According to the American Heart Association, a low-fat, high-fiber diet can reduce LDL ("bad") cholesterol levels an average of 10 percent to 15 percent. You may benefit most if you have borderline to undesirable cholesterol levels. (See "What do your cholesterol and triglyceride levels mean?" on page 24.)

What do your cholesterol and triglyceride levels mean?

To evaluate your risk of coronary artery disease, have your cholesterol and triglyceride levels measured at least every 5 years. If your values are not within desirable ranges, your doctor may advise more frequent measurements.

As you compare your numbers with these values, remember that numbers alone don't tell the whole story. Ask your doctor to interpret your test results.

	Your level*		
	Desirable	Borderline	Undesirable
Total cholesterol	Below 200	200 to 239	240 and above
LDL cholesterol	Below 130	130 to 159	160 and above
HDL cholesterol	Above 45	40 to 45	Below 40
Triglycerides	Below 150	150 to 199	200 and above

*Levels are given in milligrams of cholesterol per deciliter (mg/dL) of blood and apply to adults age 20 and older. If you have coronary artery disease, diabetes or multiple coronary artery disease risk factors, desirable values for total and LDL cholesterol are lower — LDL should be at or below 100 mg/dL.

Food better than supplements

The best way to get your fiber is from food rather than commercial fiber supplements. Supplements don't provide the nutrients found in high-fiber foods. In addition, they cost more.

Fiber supplements (Metamucil, Fibercon, Effer-syllium and others) are generally recommended if you're bothered by constipation but have trouble eating whole grains, beans and other high-fiber foods. Most supplements come in powder form that you mix with water and drink. But some are also available as biscuits, wafers, tablets or granules. When you increase your fiber intake, do it gradually and drink adequate fluids.

Fiber figures

For cholesterol-lowering benefits, aim for 5 to 9 grams of soluble fiber. To prevent constipation and diverticulosis and possibily reduce your risk of colon cancer, try to eat 25 to 30 grams of dietary fiber daily.

Food	Serving size	Total fiber (grams)	Soluble fiber (grams)
Kidney beans, cooked	1/2 cup	6.9	2.8
Black beans, cooked	1/2 cup	6.1	2.4
Apricots, with skin	4 small	3.5	1.8
Parsnips	1/2 cup	3.3	1.8
Turnips	1/2 cup	4.8	1.7
Brussels sprouts	1/2 cup	3.5	1.4
Broccoli, cooked	1/2 cup	2.6	1.1
Orange	1 medium	2.9	1.8
Apple, with skin	1 medium	3.6	1.2
Oatmeal, dry	1/3 cup	2.8	1.3

Strategy 6:
Eat more foods with antioxidants

Oxygen damage (oxidation) to your cells may be partly responsible for the effects of aging and certain diseases. Oxidation is a normal chemical process that causes cells in your arteries to more easily absorb fats and LDL ("bad") cholesterol. Over time, oxidation can speed the buildup of plaques and lead to obstruction in your arteries. Antioxidants that occur naturally in your body and certain foods may block some of this damage.

Food is the best source

Eating plenty of fruits and vegetables is the best way to consume antioxidants. Fruits and vegetables also contain soluble fiber and possibly other beneficial substances that have yet to be discovered.

If you rely on supplements to provide antioxidants, you may be missing the type and combination of substances only foods can provide.

Get your B vitamins

In addition to antioxidants, folate (vitamin B-9) has been shown to work with vitamin B-6 and vitamin B-12 to reduce blood levels of homocysteine, an amino acid. Elevated homocysteine levels can increase your risk of heart attack and stroke. Folate food sources include citrus fruits, beans, nuts, seeds, liver, dark green leafy vegetables and fortified grain products. A healthy person trying to lower the risk of cardiovascular disease should be able to get sufficient B vitamins from foods. If you have cardiovascular disease, get advice about folate (folic acid), B-6 and B-12 vitamin supplements from your doctor or dietitian.

Researchers also suspect protection may stem from a variety of substances working together rather than from isolated nutrients or substances as contained in supplements. The benefits of antioxidant supplements are unproven and taking them can be risky (see below).

Should you take antioxidant supplements?

Results of several studies now show that fruits, vegetables and whole grains that contain anti-oxidants and other nutrients may lower your risk of cardiovascular disease. But it's still unclear whether antioxidant supplements, taken as vita-min pills, have a similar benefit. As a result, the American Heart Association doesn't recommend antioxidant vitamin pills for the general public.

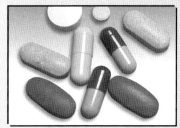

Antioxidants — including vitamins C, E and beta carotene (a form of vita-min A) — have potential health-promoting properties because they counteract oxidants, which many researchers believe play an important role in causing ath-erosclerosis.

Foods high in vitamins C, E, or beta carotene are usually low in saturated fat and cholesterol and high in fiber — characteristics that may reduce your risk of cardiovascular disease and stroke. But avoid beta carotene supplements. Recent studies show that these supplements offer no protection against heart disease, and they may pose a serious health risk for smokers and former smokers.

In contrast to earlier studies, recent studies show little benefit from vitamin E supplements in preventing heart disease or for use by high-risk heart patients. A small study (160 people) reported in the *New England Journal of Medicine* in 2001 indicates that vitamin E might interfere with cholesterol-lowering medica-tions, but more research is needed to confirm this.

If you take a blood-thinning medication such as warfarin (Coumadin, Panwarfin), large amounts of vitamin E can affect blood clotting. When it comes to preventing heart disease, any benefits from vitamin E supplements are much less than you get from exercising, eating a healthy diet and managing other risk factors, such as high blood pressure and high cholesterol.

Strategy 7:
Watch your blood pressure

High blood pressure is a major risk factor for heart attack and stroke. So it's important to have your blood pressure checked at least every 2 years or more often, depending on your medical status, family history and other risk factors. If you already have high blood pressure, you can monitor it at home — blood pressure monitors are available at medical supply stores and in many pharmacies.

For years, as long as your blood pressure was below the cutoff for being high, it was considered OK. That's not true anymore. Doctors now know that high-normal blood pressure (see chart below) often leads to high blood pressure, and high-normal blood pressure may increase your risk of cardiovascular disease.

If you're in the high-normal range or above, it's especially important to take steps to lower

Your blood pressure measurement*

	Systolic (top number)	Diastolic (bottom number)
Optimal**	120 or less	80 or less
Normal	Less than 130	Less than 85
High-normal	130 to 139	85 to 89
High (hypertension)	140 or higher	90 or higher

*Source: National Institutes of Health, 1997. Numbers are expressed in millimeters of mercury (mm Hg) and based on an average of two or more readings taken at each of two or more visits after a baseline measurement.

**Optimal means the preferred range in terms of cardiovascular risk. Unusually low readings should be evaluated.

your blood pressure to prevent cardiovascular disease. The strategies in this booklet are a good start. Many people don't make changes in their lifestyle until after their blood pressure becomes too high. But high blood pressure isn't always easy to control and it means a higher risk of a heart attack or stroke.

Ask your doctor how often you need your blood pressure checked. If your blood pressure remains consistently elevated, your doctor may recommend medication to help lower it.

Alcohol: Benefits and risks

Studies suggest that moderate amounts of alcohol can increase levels of protective HDL ("good") cholesterol and reduce your risk of heart disease. Despite these benefits, it's important to look at the risks of alcohol on an individual basis.

Excessive amounts of alcohol can raise blood pressure and damage organs, especially the liver. Heavy drinking also increases the risk of death from all causes, including cancer and hemorrhagic stroke (stroke caused by leaking or ruptured blood vessels). Even moderate amounts of alcohol can interfere with sleep, bring on headaches, cause gastritis and heartburn, and complicate depression.

Alcohol and high blood pressure

Reducing alcohol consumption can reduce your blood pressure. Heavy drinkers who cut back to moderate alcohol consumption can lower their systolic blood pressure by about 5 mm Hg and their diastolic pressure by about 3 mm Hg.

Combining a nutritious diet with reduced alcohol use can produce an even larger reduction in blood pressure. That's because people who consume too much alcohol generally don't get adequate nutrients that help control blood pressure, such as potassium, calcium and magnesium. Alcohol can also interfere with the effectiveness of some blood pressure medications and increase their side effects.

Moderation is key

The bottom line is, if you drink, do so in moderation. The Dietary Guidelines for Americans defines moderate drinking as no more than one drink a day for non-pregnant women or anyone 65 or older and no more than two drinks a day for men. One drink is 12 ounces of regular beer (150 calories), or 5 ounces of wine (100 calories), or 1.5 ounces of 80-proof distilled spirits (100 calories).

Strategy 8:
Manage stress

Little research is available that examines the impact of psychological stress on the development of cardiovascular disease. Part of the problem is that stress is a difficult concept to quantify and define. What you may find stressful, another person may find invigorating.

Although more research is needed, many cardiac rehabilitation programs use stress management as a valuable tool.

How stress affects your heart

Generally, stress is what you feel when the demands on your life exceed your ability to meet those demands. During acute stress, your body releases the hormones adrenaline and cortisol to help combat trauma or a tense situation.

Your heart beats faster, breathing quickens and blood pressure rises. You're also more susceptible to angina (a type of chest pain) and heart rhythm irregularities.

In some people, these reactions can be so dramatic that rises in blood pressure and heart rate are extreme. If stress persists, increased blood clotting as a result of the stress response can put you at risk of a heart attack or stroke.

Stress-relieving steps

Take common clues to stress — headaches, indigestion, sleeplessness and sweaty palms — seriously. Learn to manage stress using these techniques:

• *Change the factors you can* — You may not be able to walk away from a stressful job or home situation, but you can develop new responses to defuse anger or conflict. You can also learn to manage your time better by using several techniques — from delegating household responsibilities to just saying no.

• *Exercise regularly* — The natural decrease in adrenaline production after exercise may counteract the stress response. People who are physically fit handle stress better.

• *Relax* — Learning techniques such as guided imagery, meditation, muscle relaxation and relaxed breathing can help you relax. Your goal is to lower your heart rate and blood pressure while reducing muscle tension.

You can also focus on hobbies or activities you find calming, such as reading or playing with your dog.

• *Find a friend* — From dealing with cancer to coping with a troubled relationship, social support can help reduce stress and prolong life.

• *Recognize when you need help* — If stress is keeping you from work or activities, talk to your doctor or a specialist in behavioral medicine. Behavior therapy is one approach that can help you gain control over your symptoms.

Live healthy, live well

Adopting these eight strategies may seem like a daunting task. But if you make a commitment and proceed step by step, reducing your risk of a heart attack or stroke becomes a realistic goal.

As you improve your lifestyle, each step complements and builds on another. Limiting fat and cholesterol naturally leads to eating more fruits and vegetables. This boosts fiber and antioxidants, while helping control your weight. Regular exercise also contributes to a healthy weight and relieves stress.

Maintaining a healthy weight can lower blood pressure and improve blood sugar control. Monitoring your blood pressure and not smoking complete the picture of healthy living.

A healthy diet and active lifestyle aren't always enough to protect you from a heart attack or stroke. You still may need medication or other medical intervention.

But your diet and lifestyle are two areas only you control. And whether they prevent health problems or improve treatment of an illness, they're key determinants of your health and quality of life.

Stressed? Catch your breath

This quick exercise helps you learn to relax your breathing. When you're faced with a stressful situation, it can have an immediate calming effect:

1. Inhale slowly through your nose, counting to four. Imagine the inhaled, warm air flowing to all parts of your body.

2. Pause.

3. Exhale slowly through your mouth, again counting to four. Imagine the tension flowing out.

4. Pause, then begin again. Repeat several times.

GLOSSARY

Coronary artery disease: The narrowing of the arteries that serve your heart.

Cortisol: A naturally produced hormone that plays a role in a variety of body functions, including metabolism, immune function and stress response.

Isoflavones: Plant hormones that may help lower cholesterol levels. Found in most soy products.

Legume: A fruit or seed of leguminous plants such as peas or beans.

Nicotine: A highly addictive, poisonous alkaloid that is the chief active ingredient of tobacco.

Omega-3 fatty acids: A type of polyunsaturated fatty acid found mainly in cold-water fish. They seem to promote a number of factors that help prevent cardiovascular disease.

Phytoestrogens: Plant hormones that may help lower cholesterol. Found in most soy products.

Triglycerides: A form of fat that the body makes from excess calories.

Atherosclerosis, 5, 6, 10

Body mass index, 18, 20-22

Cigarette substitutes, 9
Coronary artery disease, 4-5, 24

Eating guide, 12-13

Fats
   monounsaturated, 11, 14
   polyunsaturated, 10, 14
   saturated, 11, 14
Fiber foods, 25

Obesity-related risk measurement, 22
Omega-3 fatty acids, 10
Oxidation, 26

Soy, 14
Stress reduction, 30-32
   through breathing, 32

DATE DUE

GAYLORD 234

PRINTED IN U.S.A.